DIRTY TALK

SECRETS

All the Best Practices of Dirty Talking. Sexual Fantasies, Orgasmic Pleasure, Phone Sex and Hundreds of the Right Phrases to Get Confidence with Your Partner and Fulfill Your Sex Life

Sally Meyer

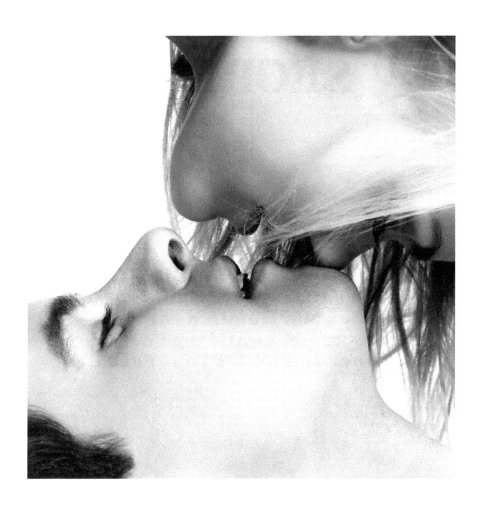

The information in the following pages is broadly considered a truthful and accurate account of facts and as such, any inattention, use, or misuse of the information in question by the reader will render any resulting actions solely under their purview. There are no scenarios in which the publisher or the original author of this work can be in any fashion deemed liable for any hardship or damages that may befall them after undertaking information described herein.

Additionally, the information in the following pages is intended only for informational purposes and should thus be thought of as universal. As befitting its nature, it is presented without assurance regarding its prolonged validity or interim quality. Trademarks that are mentioned are done without written consent and can in no way be considered an endorsement from the trademark holder.

Table of Contents

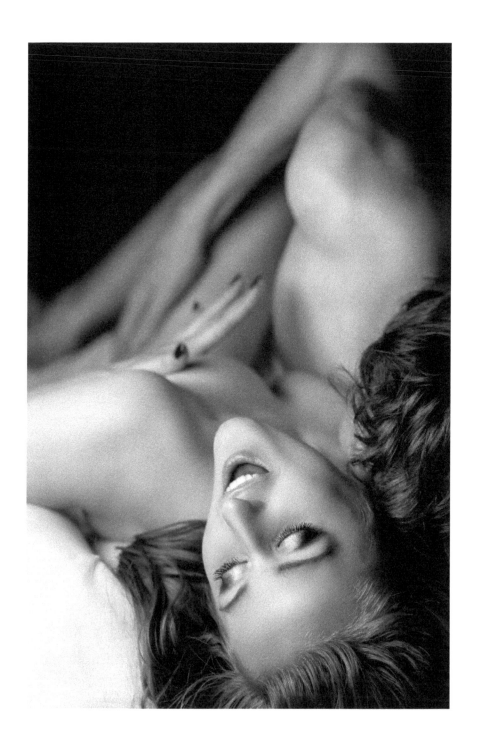

Introduction

Dirty talk is a bedroom language that we use to communicate our wants and needs.

Sometimes it is even used to convey a thought or used as a compliment.

There isn't one way to define dirty talk because it's different for all couples.

Dirty talk, also known as sexy talk, is a sexual game that uses sexual or sensual phrases to stimulate the partner's passion and pleasure and themselves through words during sex.

Words can stimulate their main senses and their partner's main senses, including touch, sight, and sound.

Even if it sounds intimidating at the moment, if you learn to talk dirty and feel more comfortable with it, you and your husband will both develop your form of conversation in the bedroom, taking you both to the limit.

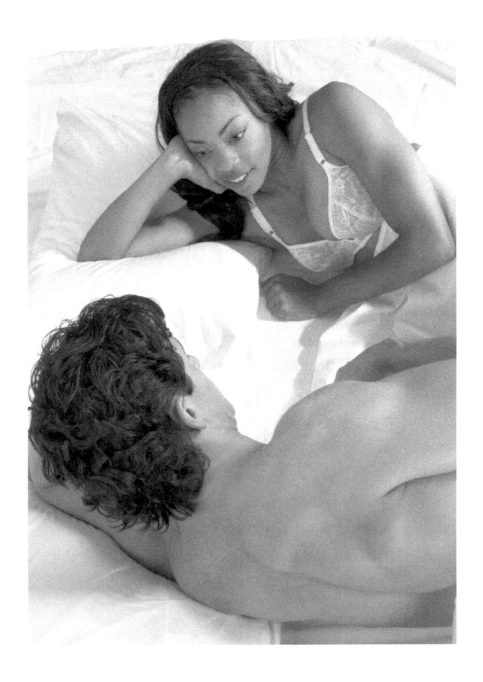

Chapter 1. Most Common Mistakes to Avoid in Dirty Talk:

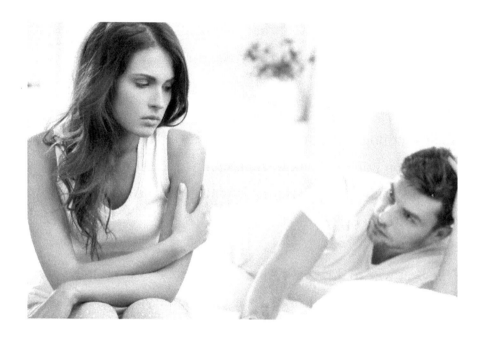

Women's magazines and blogs provide us with some very important information we can't find elsewhere. We show ideas and perspectives that help people understand and cope with or satisfy them. Many women still face the shame they try to speak dirty the first couple of times.

Your man may want to speak as dirty as you do, but someone should still make the first move. It's not so hard to live it up in the bedroom. You just need some tips. Here are a few do's, and you won't find the dirty talk helpful.

The Do's: -Tell him how large it is. Men are complementary suckers. Make his results, skills, and body feel great. This ought to go together with what he ought to do. You should tell him what to do, how to satisfy you, and how to make you feel more dirty talk.

Like anything else, you have to establish sexual confidence-before you hop into bed. It can include sex, pre-play flirting, and wordplay. The good thing is that it sets the tempo and tone for the future.

The best way to dirty talk and naturally lets it flow to tell your guy how you feel. Telling him how awesome you feel inside–that's a good way to begin.

This kind of dirty talk can be a straightforward one-" Yes! "Or it may be" I feel so good "or" yes, I like it, I love it! But foolishness depends on how open and free you and your husband are. Although building trust takes time, you can eventually.

Don't try too hard or overdo it. Don't overdo it. What you saw in porn stars may seem plausible, but if you yell all of the dirty phrases you can imagine, it spoils the mood. It's better to keep it easy, but truthful than to ruin the mood.

Don't keep it up if it isn't your friend. Here sexing and word playing is critical before pre-playing. You can say if your man is playing along or resisting.

Understand what dirty speech is, perhaps you need a guide like an eBook with everything you need to know about dirty talk. Do a little findings and find the best instruction manual to guide you from the first steps to dirty speech.

Dirty talk during sex is something everybody hasn't done before. Although a majority of us want to try it - even to fantasize, very few do.

We all know sex is an adventure, but it can also be a monotonous and dull adventure if partners do not explore new frontiers. Dirty talk will change your sexual life for the better, but you can do some crucial things and don't have to do to keep your experience meaningful.

Your friend may want to speak as dirty as you do, but you can't rekindle things unless you try. You must start slowly; not only yell all kinds of naughty things that first come to mind.

It is best to start by quietly whispering in your partner's ears, let him know what you want them to do or say and observe their answer. You will take it as an indication to say or do something. The first time is always a little tough, but one of you will take the initiative to roll the ball.

Take into account the idea of dirty talking for a few months and get to know your partner first and what kind of stuff they want.

I proposed that I spoke to my boyfriend dirty for the third month of our marriage, and to my surprise, it was just the sort of thing in which he was. Do not start dirty talking on your first night because it could turn off for some people and could be disrespectful.

The practice is required to perfect dirty talk. Only through experience do you know what your partner wants to hear, what words or phrases repel him or her, and what physical acts should be followed by what you say to each other.

It is also important to remember that dirty talk during sex may not be for everyone. My friend Lisa, who was a reserved Christian man, once told me that she tried to dirty talk at bed with her husband to spice up things but unfortunately, that had the contrary effect and caused him to immediately lose his erection.

Not only did it lead to an unpleasant circumstance, but it also led to it being called an unnecessary derogatory term. The argument here is that you must know the person with whom you are and be confident enough if you are dirty, talking, or not.

Nothing can go wrong with talking dirty, right? Wrong! As mentioned earlier, spewing a string of vulgar or profane words is not what dirty talk is in the context of sexual relationships.

The words you say don't matter as much as how and when you say them. You want to avoid coming off a tat; talking dirty is not synonymous with the ramblings in porn movies. Unlike porn, getting your erotic talk right can increase the love and affection you share with your partner. And even if you are in a casual relationship or having a one-night stand, you can still use dirty talk correctly to increase your sex experience.

Let us quickly consider some of the things that can go wrong with dirty talk.

Avoid These Dirty Talk Mistakes

Going full steam ahead

Even if your partner loves talking dirty, jumping into it with all the filthy words you can come up with is not the best way to go. Start slowly with innocent or tame words and phrases. As your foreplay and feeling of ecstasy increases, you can ease into the flow of stronger terms and graphic descriptions. Baby steps are always crucial when dealing with emotions and feelings.

Talking non-stop

Porn stars may keep talking dirty throughout sex, but that is just an act. Bringing that into your bedroom may give your partner a different opinion about you, whether they are casual partners or you are in a long-term relationship with them.

There is nothing wrong with saying only a handful of phrases throughout sex. Only talk when you want to talk. Remember, a large part of talking dirty reacts to what you feel and not just putting up an act.

Too much profanity

It may be called "dirty," but that doesn't mean every statement must be loaded with curse words and profanity. Suppose you always use derogatory terms when referring to your partner during sex and don't include loving, kind, and appreciative words in your dirty talks.

In that case, your partner may begin to think you see them in that light. It is not a mistake to adhere to the saying; too much of everything is bad. I highly recommend using profanity or curse words like the icing on your sex cake, and not the main ingredient.

Laughing at your partner's remark

It is okay to introduce humor in sex. It is equally okay to have hearty laughs together as part of foreplay or after sex. But it is not okay to laugh at your partner's remark, even if they get their lines wrong. You may hurt their ego or ruin their mood, especially if they are new to dirty talk or trying to break out of their shell and overcome shyness.

Shaming your partner's body parts or degrading their performance

If you must talk about your partner's body, let your sex talks focus on the things you like about them. If you find nothing to appreciate in their body (such as in the case of a one-night stand), do not comment on their body parts, especially intimate ones.

Instead, focus only on how you feel, what you want them to do, or what you want to do. Making belittling remarks in the guise of profanity may turn your partner off completely.

Avoid it by all means. Making insane remarks such as, "I want to crush your stupid pussy," or "Can't you fuck me any harder?" are thoughtless forms of verbal abuse and shouldn't be confused with dirty talk. People have insecurities about their bodies and sexual performances. Don't be insensitive to these insecurities and make degrading remarks about their body or performance.

Being tentative

You will turn off the heat if you sound unsure when you speak. For example, when you say, "You like it when I do that, don't you?" make it sound like a statement rather than a question.

While it can be very sexy to speak in low tones, it doesn't mean you can't sound confident. When you play a submissive role, it is okay to sound pleasing to your partner and even pretend to beg (yes, submissive roles require assuming a weak position).

But a dominant role is authoritative in many ways. You can't play both parts at the same time. Tailor your dirty talk to suit one role at a time.

Being repetitive

It becomes boring after a while if you always repeat the same line. If you run out of ideas on what to say, stick to moaning and using body language.

Avoid sounding like a broken record. Every sex act is different, and even if you can't find entirely new phrases to use, creatively tweak the ones already know. When you keep your partner guessing your next naughty line, it can build sexual anticipation and make the mood last longer.

Forcing it

The goal of talking dirty is to increase sexual enjoyment. If something you are saying isn't working, stop and try something else. Don't force a line that just isn't working, or else you will begin to sound like a phony. If you've tried a few times, and your creative juices are not just flowing, give it a rest and focus on allowing your other bodily juices to flow.

Let your partner do the talking or simply enjoy silent sex for that moment. There is always another time to put your dirty talking skills into action.

Giving up too soon

So, you've tried a few times, and it seems you are not cut out for this type of erotic expression. The worst mistake is to give up the idea entirely. Patience and communication are vital to developing this skill. It is not easy for many people (not just you) to verbalize their deepest feelings, especially when those feelings are intimate or sexual. To make it even worse, it is more difficult to express such sexual desires using suggestive and graphic terms. It takes a lot of practice and explorative investigation to get this right. However, the benefits are worth all the effort.

Dismissing the use of protection

This is particularly for people in a casual relationship or for couples who are not ready to make babies. No matter how horny you get from hearing all the naughty sex talks, insist on using protection.

Saying things like, "Now, let's slip a condom over this gorgeous cock/penis," should do it. Consider the type of message you are silently passing to a casual partner if you are not bothered whether they use protection or not. Apart from pregnancy, sexually transmitted diseases can be avoided through the use of protection.

Chapter 2.
Perfect Practice

It is time to put what you've learned so far into practice. This chapter contains exercises designed to:

1. Reduce any awkward feeling beginners to dirty talk may experience.

2. Help you discover the types of erotic words that are most comfortable for you.

3. Increase your comfortability with hearing and saying gross words during foreplay and sex.

4. Stimulate yourself to come up with your unique love talks and phrases.

I strongly recommend completing the first two exercises before attempting the rest in any order you choose.

Exercise 1: Build a List of "Safe Erotic Phrases"

Erotic talk can be challenging for many people, especially if you don't know the words to use. This exercise helps you to choose "safe erotic phrases" that are not vulgar but very titillating.

Choose phrases that are at your tolerance level. You and your partner don't have to use words and phrases you both consider off-limits. You can complete this exercise alone and ask your partner to do the same, or you can do it together.

1. Get a pen and paper.

2. Make a list of phrases and words you find comfortable and sexually arousing. For example:

· "I can't wait to feel your hands all over my body."

· "I've been fantasizing about you inside me all day."

· "Touch me here on my (body part) softly."

· "Your (body part) feels so delicious."

· "Go slower/faster."

· "Be gentle/rough with me tonight."

· "Go on your knees and beg for it."

· "I love your (body part) when you (action)."

· "Kiss my (body part) with your warm lips."

· "Keep doing that... yes, that's the spot."

3. Now, say them out loud to yourself and gauge your mood as you hear yourself say these words. Do they make you horny? Or do they sound repulsive? Exclude any phrase that turns you off.

4. When you are done with your list, exchange them with your partner.

Exercise 2: Make an "Off-Limits" List

Since everyone has a different view of what is offensive, it is important to let your partner know your offensive definition. This exercise helps you and your partner know each other's off-limits words. You need to be truthful when you do this exercise. Don't settle for a term just to make your partner happy. Setting personal boundaries is crucial for your happiness and sexual satisfaction.

1. Begin by writing down a list of off-limits words and phrases. For example:

· Cum, slut, fuck, cock, pussy, dick, cunt, whore, bitch, etc.

· Good girl, good boy, little girl, slave, daddy, prisoner, and so on.

2. You don't have to explain why you find these phrases or words offensive (unless if you choose to). Simply let your partner know that these phrases turn you off or you find them disgusting.

3. Go through the examples of dirty talk in this book to find more words and phrases you consider offensive. Add them to your list.

4. Exchange this list with your partner. You can send your list to your partner through text or email and get them to do the same.

Exercise 3: Working Your Way Up to "Dirty" Words

In this exercise, you will write down short phrases that you find comfortable. They don't have to be vulgar or contain profanity at first. You are going to work your way from seemingly innocent terms to graphic terms. Here's what to do:

1. Get a pen and paper.

2. Write down a sensual or romantic phrase you think you can comfortably say during foreplay or sex. For example, "Let's make love."

3. Think of another way of saying that phrase such that it doesn't lose its meaning and yet, not too difficult for you to say. For example, you can go from sounding romantic to using official terms. "Let's make love" could easily become, "Let's have sex."

4. Now tweak the phrase a bit to sound more street-like. For example, "Let's shag."

5. Finally, find a graphic term that can convey the same meaning. For example, "Let's fuck!"

You don't have to use the graphic or vulgar term with your partner just yet.

Keep on building your list of comfortable vulgar words and saying them to yourself when you are alone. You can look in the mirror while you practice.

Practice switching from sensual to official-sounding terms with your partner for a while. Gradually introduce street slangs. And when you think you can use graphic words without feeling like dying, go ahead and use them with your partner.

Exercise 4: Sound and Whispers

It is easy to think that talking dirty usually means talking like a porn star – screaming profanity at the top of your voice during foreplay and sex. You don't have to wake the kids or disturb your neighbors with your gross talks. One of the most effective ways to say these things is by softly whispering them. This exercise will help you perfect your whispering skills to get your partner all fired up and ready to go!

1. You will need your partner for this exercise. Get comfortable beside them.

2. Breathe in deeply and let your body relax.

3. Think of something sensual and connect with that feeling.

4. Make a low sound – moan, groan, or even a soft giggle.

5. Inhale a bit loudly and when you exhale, let the air out of your mouth with a soft moaning sound.

6. Now, softly whisper one of your practiced phrases in your partner's ears. You don't have to be coherent or loud. It doesn't matter what you say, so long as you whisper it, it will sound sexier.

The fainter and sexier your voice, the closer they'll have to listen. This removes any awkwardness you may feel from hearing yourself say filthy things. And even if you get a few words wrong, it wouldn't be so apparent since you are only whispering.

The tingling sensation your partner feels in their spine as your breath and words softly caress their ears increases the sexual effects of your words.

7. You can stop when you've practiced this exercise for a few minutes. Laugh about it or consider it as foreplay. It is okay if things "get out of hand" during the exercise, and you end up

having hot, steamy sex. It only goes to show that you used your sounds and whispers effectively.

Exercise 5: Stay in Character

This exercise helps to build your sexual confidence using role-play. You will need your partner and a timer for this exercise.

1. Think of a character that is completely different from you in real-life. If your partner likes, they can also choose a different character or simply watch your performance.

For example, a naughty teacher, a vile warder, a sex-starved nurse or doctor, and so on. Whichever role you choose, your partner can play a role that goes with it. For example, teacher/student, warder/prisoner, nurse/patient or doctor/patient.

2. Set a stop clock for five minutes (you can increase when you get the hang of this).

3. Now, talk like the character you have chosen for the next five minutes or whatever time you have set. Remember to stay in character. Talk like a naughty teacher or sex-starved nurse would (or whatever role you have chosen).

4. You don't have to screen out words that you consider offensive when playing your character's role. After all, it is your character talking and not you. So, don't feel shy or refrain from saying curse words or using profanity if it suits your character.

5. When your timer goes off, step out of character, and ask your partner for feedback. If you both participated in the role-play, you should also provide your partner with feedback.

6. Remember to make this exercise as fun as you can. Think of it as foreplay.

Exercise 6: Rehearse and Record

This works especially well for improving your erotic talks on the phone. For this exercise, you will need a recorder to record what you say. You can use the audio recorder on your smartphone for this.

1. Get comfortable on your bed, preferably where you will not be disturbed for about five to twenty minutes.

2. Pretend that you are talking with your partner on the phone and want to initiate phone sex. It is helpful to hold your phone

to your ear to give you a sense of actually talking to someone on the other end.

3. Press record and begin talking. Talk and imagine that your partner is responding to what you say. Let your imagination run wild and say exactly what you feel and want. Remember, no one is watching or listening, so don't be shy or reserved.

4. It is possible to get very aroused during this exercise. But if you feel nothing, it is still okay. The important thing is to go with your imagination flow and express what is on your mind as if you are having phone sex.

5. Stop the recording when you are done talking. Now playback your solo conversation and learn how you sound when you are not worried about what anyone thinks. This is exactly how you want to be sounding when you are having actual phone sex.

6. Also, listen to uncover areas where you think you could improve.

Exercise 7: Codify Your Sex Talk

Sometimes, you may find it awkward or embarrassing to use too strong words, especially if you are new to the concept of using gross bedroom language. At other times, you may find that you are stuck with only a few overused or outdated phrases. To avoid these situations, it is a good idea to develop some of your unique codes or phrases that tell your partner what you want to say without actually saying them.

To do this:

1. Get a pen and paper.

2. Think of potential awkward statements and write them down. For example:

· "I want to ride your cock."

· "Suck my hard cock while I lick your wet cunt."

· "I need your warm, sexy mouth around my hard dick."

3. Think of a phrase that can replace these potentially embarrassing words and write them beside the first statements. Using the above examples:

· "I want to ride your cock," could become, "My turn."

· "Suck my hard cock while I lick your wet cunt," could become, "It's time for my favorite thing."

· "I need your warm, sexy mouth around my hard dick," could become, "Please me."

4. When you have put down as many potentially embarrassing statements as you can think of, show you partner your list and ask them to write theirs and share with you.

5. Even when you get comfortable talking dirty, you could turn this into a game where you both come up with different codes that are unique to two of you. You could have a sexual conversation in the presence of people without them knowing what you are up to. This is a cool way to keep your things spiced up between you.

Exercise 8: Dirty Talks Just for Fun

This exercise is great if you have a partner that is shy or not open to sex talks.

1. Find a time and place where you are both relaxed, but not necessarily in the mood for having sex.

2. Tell your partner that you want to say a few erotic phrases/words to them and need them to rate how sexy or filthy they think the phrases/words are. You can tell them to rate the statements using a scale of 0 to 10 or anything suitable.

3. Start with short "innocent" phrases and gauge their response.

4. If they don't seem interested, don't push them or force it. Give it a rest and bring it up at another time when they seem to be more relaxed.

5. If they seem interested, take it up a notch. You can even ask them to give you some suggestions. For example, "Would you prefer me to say 'vagina' or 'pussy'?" Or "Does 'cock' and 'cum' sound too strong for you? Perhaps I should stick to 'penis,' what do you think?"

6. No matter the positive response you get from a shy partner, remember to always keep this exercise short. Don't over flog it, or else you may push them too hard too soon.

Extra Tips to Help a Shy Partner Open to Erotic Talk

You may have no qualms vocalizing your thoughts, feelings, and requests before, during, and after sex, but you may be stuck with a partner that is too shy to utter any word apart from occasional moans.

The following tips can help them adjust and become more open to expressing themselves. Always remember that we are all different.

Not everyone enjoys saying what they want or what they want to do during sex. So be patient with your partner if they are the shy type.

Encourage Them to Text It

You don't have to directly ask them to text you something erotic or filthy.

You could send them a text about what you intend to do with them later in the day and ask if it's okay or they'll like to make some adjustments.

For example, "You, me, candlelight dinner, 8 pm, my place. A hot bath, and then sex in the shower. Your thoughts?"

Allowing your partner to text you back, their thoughts create room for them to loosen up and be a bit more expressive. Also, remember to keep your questions open-ended when you talk dirty to them.

Chapter 3. Sex Phone

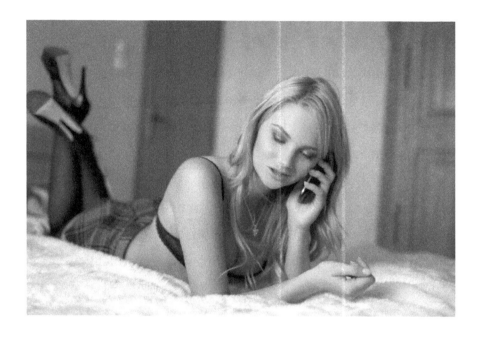

Whether your partner lives with you or is in a long-distance relationship, you can take advantage of technology to spice up your sex life with phone sex.

Phone sex can also work for you if you don't want to have other forms of sex with your partner just yet, or if you simply want to try something new. Although the idea of having phone sex can be exciting, it may be awkward when you want to try it out for the first time.

Having physical sex or even masturbating alone is a lot easier because no one else is aware of what you are doing. But having to possibly masturbate (it's not compulsory to do so) with another person hearing and maybe even seeing you through video requires a different level of boldness.

To make phone sex a great and sexually exciting experience, you need to give up being self-conscious and intentionally allow yourself to respond to the sounds and sight coming to you from the other end.

Also, remember to have a conversation instead of a monologue. Phone sex is not a hypnotic session. Both partners should share what they are doing, imagining, and feeling.

Sex on Call

The process

Plan ahead: Spontaneity is great when it comes to sex, but sometimes you may call your partner at the wrong time. To avoid this, set a date and time that is most convenient for both of you.

If you are in the mood for sex while your partner is having a bad day, calling them at that time may ruin your mood. Also, if your partner is the shy type, it may be a good idea to get their minds prepared on time before you pounce on them with your sexy talk on the phone.

Put yourself in the mood: Feeling awkward or tensed before your call will probably ruin the mood. Do what you need to do to get in the mood before the call. You can have a glass of wine, watch short porn, read a romance or porn novel, or even dancing.

Dressing sexily and lying down for a while can also put you in a sexy mood. You can also dim the lights, play your favorite soft music, bring out some sex toys (if you use them), and gently caressing yourself before making the call.

Make the call: There is no one correct format for phone sex. However, once your partner is on the phone with you, it is better to start slowly.

Talk about other things for a few minutes before gradually broaching the subject of sex. Make your voice soft, low, and don't be afraid to moan. You can use heavy breathing too, as long as it comes naturally. Don't force yourself to sound sexy.

Talk about easy things: You don't have to directly bring up sex, even if both of you know the call is about sex. Ease into phone sex with simple topics that can easily spiral into hot sex. The following writings will give you an idea of how to do this.

1. What are you wearing?

2. It's cold here. I wish you were here.

3. This bed is just too wide for me alone.

4. I'm lying on your side of the bed and playing with my hair.

5. I wish you were here beside me.

6. Tell me what you are doing with your hands?

7. Tell me what you would have done to me if I were there with you now.

Talk dirty: Once the mood is right, escalate into dirty talk. Since they are not physically with you, your dirty talk will have to be descriptive. Both of you can describe:

What you are doing: give your partner a vivid description of how and where you are touching yourself, how you look, what you are playing with, and so on. You can say things such as:

1. I'm playing with that whip you bought from an adult store for our first role play.

2. My fingers are teasing my cock as we speak.

3. I'm touching my tits, and my nipples are so hard.

4. I'm playing with my undies... they are coming off soon.

5. I'm getting wet and horny.

6. I enjoy listening to your sexy voice. It's making me hard/wet.

7. I'm running my fingers through my hair.

8. I'm jerking off to the sound of your sexy moan.

What you are imagining: Tell your partner something you remember from one of your great sex you had, what you would have loved to be doing with them, or what you would want them to do to you. For example:

1. I'd like to hug you real close and feel the warmth of your soft skin.

2. I'd like to kiss your neck, lips, and tits ever so softly.

3. Remember how you took me from behind the last night we had together? Now, take me again!

4. I'm touching myself and thinking how great your hands feel all over me.

5. Touch your clit and feel my warm breath on your pussy.

6. I can imagine how rock solid your cock will be now. I want to stroke it and suck on it with my wet lips.

7. I can tell you are soaking wet. Imagine me eating out that wet pussy.

8. Put one finger in your mouth and imagine it's my cock in there.

· How you feel: It is important to let your partner know the effect of the conversation on you. Describe how you feel physically and emotionally. You can moan loudly, scream (if you have to), or breathe deeply. Let go of all inhibitions and allow yourself to be fully expressed. You can say something such as:

1. The sound of your voice is making my heart beat faster.

2. I feel like exploding when you sound like that.

3. Say that again... please. It feels so good to hear you say that.

4. You are making me quake with that moaning sound.

5. I feel like appearing right there with you.

6. I feel sexy when you call me your little girl.

7. I feel like kissing your lips now!

8. Oh my God! I'm coming!

Masturbate if you feel like it: If you choose, you can masturbate while talking with your partner and let them listen to all your moans, or you can engage in mutual masturbation. But this is completely optional. It is okay to skip it if it doesn't feel right or appropriate.

It is also good to keep in mind that phone sex may not always end in orgasm. Only one of you may climax, or both of you may fail to climax, and that is okay.

Orgasm is not the main attraction of phone sex. However, if you have climaxed and your partner has not yet reached the orgasm, don't end the call or keep mute. Continue to describe how you feel, what you want them to do, and so on.

Finish the call: You can end the call at any time both of you choose. You must not reach orgasm before ending the call. Also, you shouldn't end the call just because you've both climaxed. You can stay on the line for as long as you both choose and talk chit chat a bit.

Talk about it afterward: Don't be shy to talk about the phone sex afterward. You can even text them how great it felt. Compliment them either on call on through text and make them know that you are looking forward to another great phone sex.

Keeping shut about it afterward may suggest that you are uncomfortable or you feel guilty.

Sex on a video call

You can take advantage of different technologies (FaceTime, Skype, Zoom, and so on) to have sex "face-to-face" over your devices. Seeing what your partner is doing, their reaction to what you are saying, and their facial expressions can add to the arousal, especially for men.

To avoid frustration and disruptions that can kill the mood, make sure that your internet signal is strong enough for video calls or simply sticking to phone sex.

Sexting

Sexting is using digital messages to convey erotic intents. Thanks to technology, people can now send naughty messages back and forth without dealing with the uneasiness that comes with saying these words face-to-face.

You can use sexting to gauge a potential partner's openness even before dating them or having sex with them. However, sexting techniques range from subtle to direct methods. It is always a nice idea to begin sexting with subtle messages that can pass as flirting.

If the other person responds positively, you can then up your game to messages that puts them in a sexy mood. Finally, you can sext messages that make them want to have sex with you so badly.

Sexting can be done using text only or inserting photos, memes, emojis, and emoticons. Get adventurous with your messages and make them unique. The following examples are just to give you an idea of what sexts look like. It will make

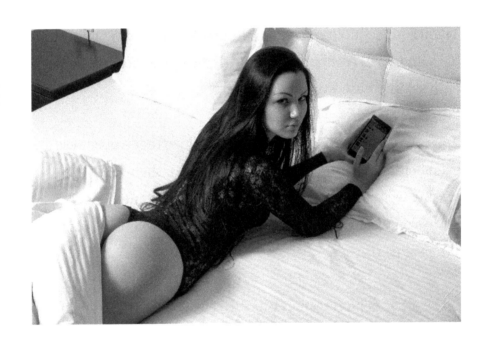

more impact if you adapt your sext to something you and your partner share or experience. For example, instead of just sending, "I can't stop thinking of your sexy ass," you can personalize it to read, "I can't stop thinking of your sexy ass in those red yoga pants." Or "Those pants hug your ass so tightly I feel like touching myself." A good sext is usually short and stimulates sexual imagination. Even when you use sexual innuendos, keep it brief. If you can make room for humor, that will be great too.

Go through the examples below and let your creative juices guide you into creating customize sext messages for your long-term partner or someone new you are trying to have sex with.

Beginner sexting examples

1. Guess what? I'm at work thinking of you and touching myself right now.

2. Your hot ass/legs dominate my thoughts all day.

3. What part of my body is your favorite?

4. I can still feel your warm lips on my cheeks.

5. I need you right now.

6. Can we do it in the shower tonight?

7. I'm soaking wet right now. Can you come over for a quickie?

8. Next time, I'll lick more places on your hot body.

9. Your cock/pussy makes me go insane.

10. You went down on me, and I lost all my senses.

11. You. Me. Under the sheets... pure heaven!

12. I love how hard you gave it to me last night. Let's make it even rougher next time.

13. I love how you take charge of my body.

14. I want you to dominate me tonight.

15. This early morning's quickie was delicious. Can we continue tonight?

16. I get goosebumps when I think of your hands in my pants / up my skirt.

17. You look so sexy and innocent when you giggle.

18. I don't feel like having my bath just yet. I love the smell of you on me.

19. Whenever you pass by, I get a boner. Can you help me fix that?

20. Let's do something freaky tonight. Got any sexy ideas?

21. I want to have dinner off of your body tonight.

22. I need your naked body on mine right now.

23. Picture this in your mind: you and me, naked under my sheets.

24. Let's have a mixed wrestling match tonight. No count-out or disqualifications. Don't worry; I'll be gentle when I slam you on the bed.

25. URGENT! Can you please help me with five synonyms for FUCK?

Advance sexting examples

1. What crazy place should we fuck next time?

2. You have no idea how hard you make me want to fuck you.

3. Your ass is so sexy. It deserves an Instagram page.

4. My dick/pussy still feels lusciously sore from yesterday's pounding. You sure know how to handle me.

5. I can still taste your sweet cum on my lips.

6. I'll like you to cum all over my tits tonight.

7. Come straight to bed after work. There's a wet pussy waiting to be fucked!

8. Three things occupied my mind all day: your sumptuous boobs, succulent lips, and wet pussy!

9. Thinking of the sound you make when you cum makes me want to cum in my pants!

10. I'll let you cum in my mouth if you let me sit on your face tonight.

Creative sexting examples

1. A sexy surprise awaits you tonight... *insert wink emoji*

2. I've been thinking of your *insert peach emoji* all day.

3. I'll love to do this tonight... *insert sex position GIF*

4. Your ass is so *insert hot/fire emoji* it makes my dick *insert raindrops/sweat droplets emoji*

5. *Insert bondage GIF* Tonight will be fun!

6. I want to *insert tongue emoji* your *insert peach emoji* right this minute.

7. Me when I saw your naked boobs last night *insert head exploding GIF*

8. *Insert eggplant emoji* Free services tonight. *insert wink emoji*

9. *Insert image of a man proposing* with a meme caption: When she says, "Cum in my mouth."

10. *Insert an image of a breathless woman or woman fanning herself* with a meme caption: When he asks, "How would you like to be fucked tonight?"

11. Tonight was exceptional. Thank you! *insert heart and worship hands emoji*

12. Meme caption: You: smooching my cock/tits. Me: *insert fainting image*

Chapter 4. Dirty talk in public

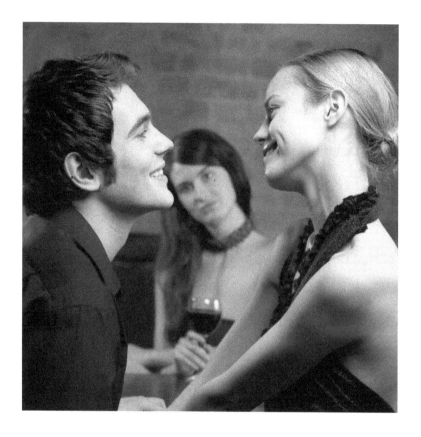

Phone texting, sex, cybersex, email... All of these are things that maintain the filthy conversation between you and your partner.

However, how about this exhibitionist side of you personally, the one which cries how poorly you need your partner, plus it is irrelevant where? You might maintain a public park, a railway station, a discount store, a financial institution, and even in the household. Maybe you've had a lot of at the x-mas party, or maybe you are all set to receive it on at the pool. In any case, might be, you can talk dirty -- and you are in public areas.

Not a problem! The best technique for talking dirty in people is to make certain nobody knows precisely what you're saying. They may imagine, convinced, but who cares? Should they don't understand without a doubt, they cannot call you on it!

When you can manage to receive your partner sexy and sexy as you're in a public atmosphere, you are certain to get some wonderful actions whenever you do arrive at a relaxing and private place.

Below are a couple of strategies to begin talking dirty in people: whisper it. The very populous, crazy dirty talk is stated using a whisper.

Say it with a sly grin and let your lips brush the fan's ear since you let them know exactly what you desire to complete in their mind later. Or that which you need them to complete for your requirements.

When it's a quick and pleasant opinion, something such as I need to fuck you," it's sufficient to have the ball rolling. Show it. Say it along with your own eyes.

Let your partner know you just want them by how you glance at them. Good dirty talk may comprise more than simply words! Make a place of appearing in the lover's tight, sexy cute butt with pride in your eyes.

Make certain that you get stuck doing this! If you would like to get right to the purpose, shed your own eyes into his crotch, linger there some time, then look back into your own eyes. Any man worth his salt will soon know exactly what that look means! Slip away.

Simply take the opportunity for you to hide out for some time and enjoy a small amount of appetite. Perhaps it is possible to discover a secluded hallway and cop a feel. Maybe you can sneak a profound French kiss as you're headed to the kitchen to match your beverage.

Whenever you do slide away, be sure that you set your feelings into words. Cause them to become clear and to the purpose. "I want to suck you off to the table" can be just a fantastic way to elevate your buff's eyebrows!

Let the body do the talking. Whenever you are standing close, brush your breasts against his spine. Let your buttocks touch. Put your arm.

Slip down your hand to an improper place today and then, however, just for an instant, before anybody else could grab onto exactly what that gloomy hand is doing. Lean over and utilize the dirty words to finish the emotional picture.

Innuendo galore! Certainly, one of the best things about the filthy conversation in people is that moment when someone says something innocent...nevertheless, you hear it within a naughty method. Dirty thoughts build, one after another.

The further cluttered your thinking will be, the more inclined you should observe the many naive comments as raunchy chances.

As an example, if someone expresses it's hot out, you could lean to a partner and say," maybe not as sexy as it will be " the dual significance won't be lost to these, and so on you'll be laughing in the most useful "naive" opinions -- and becoming switched at exactly the same moment.

Make dirty conversation in people a match the 2 of you play with together. Inform your spouse at the onset of the evening, which you're going to undoubtedly be talking dirty to him that the whole time and have him rely on the number of dirty-talk opinions they will capture.

Subsequently, slide into those naughty innuendos every chance you will get! Below are a couple of suggestions to help get this gloomy innuendo started: while at a Fourth of July party, speak to just how nicely those temples are "shooting" to the atmosphere.

Tell him just how much you want the noise of this "cannon" and inquire whether he believes they have been planning to "blow" a whole lot larger for the "orgasm" when at the shore, say that cream feels "thick and warm and creamy" like something you may think about...when you visit someone about the surfboard, mention that you'll like to become riding something hard, too.

Maybe the very thought of this something hard it which makes you wet as a sea! At a friend's party? Discuss how you adore the taste of the jello "shooters" and point out that the restroom is far a lot more than big enough for just two.

If you should be in an incredibly adventuresome mood and you also understand that your partner is a thing a little more "enjoyable," play with a match of speaking about that man at your buddy's party are the loudest in bed, or that you would love to invite for a threesome. Discussing of threesomes and other naughty tidbits

People "Whoa!" Seconds

We've mentioned how to dirty talk creates pictures in mind, images that function to direct your spouse. Speaking about what you are doing during intercourse or requesting him exactly what he wants to accomplish opens the doorway to deeper conversation.

People do a good deal of things from the heat of fire they mightn't ordinarily do, and you should immediately realize they say things that they normally wouldn't state, too.

One dream contributes to still another, yet still another, and so on, you may end up exploring land you won't ever have differently, had you never heard that this fresh foul speech. Opinions may be earned in the heat of the fire that surprises you, makes you uneasy, as well as shock you.

You could hear matters you had never anticipated, and you also could not understand just how to react.

However, before you become angry, look at this: whenever you are switched on beyond belief, how have you been thinking about that from mouthwatering? Are you aware of the small pops and sighs you simply can't appear to help? It's the same with a vibrant dream -- whether or not it's in mine, it's probably likely to be said at a certain time, however raunchy or taboo it's.

That is one of those cool ideas about mind-blowing gender: it destroys the filter that typically governs the mouth area! If a partner does feel liberated to express what for you, which you've never heard previously, make an effort to contain your shock in what's said. Remember: you hear these matters as you've accumulated the closeness between both of you personally, and discussing those dreams requires an enormous step of confidence.

When he did not hope you, then you will not hear his innermost thoughts and secrets! The simple fact he has only told you something intimate about his wants speaks volumes regarding how he feels about you.

Therefore, be thankful he can say such things! Granted, a number of dreams might be gasp-inducing. It may be something as straightforward as requesting to wear high heeled boots and fishnets at the bed.

Also it may be something as jaw-dropping as though he'd like to see one with the other woman -- or even some other guy! The graphics that your good dirty conversation paints within his mind could swell into pictures that you never imagined being there.

This is a standard development; although you could be taken aback in the beginning, it's essential to not forget this heightened familiarity is a fantastic thing. Try not to get confused by the dreams he relates.

However, does not accept these since the gospel, either. Studies indicate that ninety percent of dreams are simply that -- a dream. They're matters which turn you when you consider these; however, you may not perform in actuality, given that the ability.

Lots of men and women discuss exactly what they'd like to complete, or they could take to one afternoon; however, few chase it. The dream is normally enough. Sharing those dreams may cause amazing sex between the 2 of you.

However, it generally does not suggest he wishes to own this wonderful sex using four or three -- or even longer! If you are into the dirty conversation, then you are already pretty open-minded. Keep this receptive mind once you are in the heat of the fire and talking dreams.

Who knows? However, if the bedroom matches are over and it's only the couple at the afterglow, you could begin to wonder about what that came from the mouth area. Can he mention just how good it is to see with another guy?

Can he be really to with two ladies during sex together with him? And lord have mercy, did he mean it if he said he wished to stop by a gay strip club? You might discover some crazy objects once the inhibitions are unleashed. Below are a few chances.

How do you believe if you hear a couple of these? I would like to see you during sex with another guy. I would like to see you during sex with another lady. I would like to let my very best friend take a look. I would like one to complete me as if my cousin did me personally.

I'd like to be tied up and spanked. I would like one to visit a strip club and see you get yourself a lap dancing. I would like one to see me have a lap dancing. I would like to try out smoking buds while we put it all on.

I would like you to whip me. I would like to meet a stranger in a hotel room and have sex. I would like to dress up in your clothes.

I would like to test out women and also men. I would like to get fucked up the bum with a strap on. I'd like to inform you and cause you to call me daddy. I would like one to bark like a dog while I fuck you.

I would like to find out you decorate in leather. (or perhaps just a French maid outfit, or hooker heels, etc.) That I need to make you my sex slave. Therefore...what exactly do you think? Do some of these tricks allow you to cringe? Do some of these turn you?

Can a number of them cause you to desire to quit reading? All these are now pretty tame when compared with this huge dream world within our minds. Your man may have a really special fantasy that has quite a while to spell out. Or it may be something you've never been aware of earlier.

Again, do not judge this, and do not make an effort to show him off from that which he is simply told you. Bear in mind the dilemma of trust and just how much it required him to express the things for you.

—

Think of it as a compliment! Bear in mind: your partner probably needed a sexual past until you came across, and you also have been rounding the block several times, too. In any event, because he says it can't mean he wishes to accomplish it, and only because he said it couldn't mean he has been down the road.

It's possible to take those dreams for what they have been -- a filthy conversation between two different people at a fervent moment -- or you'll be able to ask additional questions. However, before you start, bear in mind that your fantasies. What are you ever said in the heat of fire which you'll not truly do?

Research indicates that many women think of being accepted by greater than one person, but most of them could not decide to try it. Research also demonstrates that rape is now an interest of many women's dreams, but not one of these would want it to manifest! What happens within our minds, in our private thoughts, is frequently not something which meshes together with this true to life.

This is exactly why it's referred to as a dream. If you're still determined to arrive at the underside of the dreams, be warned: don't ask if that you never desire to understand! If you'd rather never be worried about your partner's sexual history, do not inquire if certain dreams happened. He would let you know that the reality, of course, should you've got any jealousy in any way; you may turn green with jealousy and crimson with anger.

He may lie for you, which divides the closeness you've assembled, and that makes him likely to maintain his head to himself on out.

However, if you should be entirely confident in your relationship and prepared to be adventurous because he's, by all means, talk every dream that springs to mind.

There is nothing sexier than understanding what a sexual encounter your partner needs and establishing that do or may result in some intense debate -- and who knows? Some particular" whoa" moments only may result in some intense experiences you never dreamed you'd pursue!

Chapter 5.
Dirty Talk and Orgasmic Pleasure

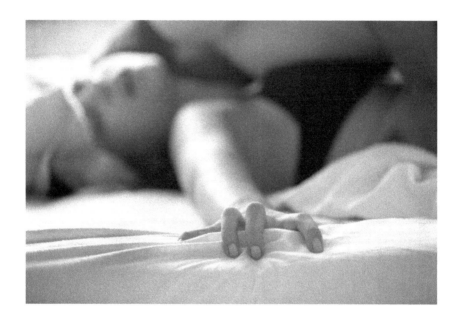

Dirty Talk Secrets for Talking Her into Orgasmic Pleasure

Dirty Talk in bed is probably the most misunderstood, underestimated, and abused form of foreplay. Make no mistake.

You can give your spouse much better orgasms during sex if you start talking DIRTY. You see, talking dirty enhances all the physical energy you do with your wife in the bedroom.

• Talk dirty to your wife while you touch her, and it will be more exciting for her.

• Talk dirty to your spouse while "taking her from behind," and she will do more.

• Talk dirty while screaming through a strong vaginal orgasm, and you will enjoy it more.

Dirty Talk is as Powerful as You Think

You are going to discover how to give your husband an orgasm on request. Basically, this ensures that his wife will come if you tell her too. Believe me when I say that it will be inspiring for you and her, and it will occur to you.

See how you do it.

You should start training your wife to be extremely sensitive to your voice and have her relate her orgasms to your dirty talk.

The next time you are with your wife, and she almost has an orgasm, say this:

• YOU: "Honey, you want to come now, right?"

• HER: "Oh, yes."

• YOU: "You come so hard for me."

• SHE: "Oh my God, yes."

(Keep saying the above until it takes a second to her coming)

Then say this right at the point as she is starting to have her orgasm

YOU: "Come for me, baby, come now, come strong for me."

What just happened is that you told her to come, and she came

Here is the Key

Do the same thing several times over a few weeks, and you will find your wife becoming more sensitive to your dirty words.

Finally, you can tell her about ORGASM ON-COMMAND, and she will do it.

If she's very aroused, wet, and ready to come, says:

"Come to me now."

And she will.

Why Do Women Like Dirty Talk?

Women love Dirty Talk because, in bed, it can convey the quality that women find extremely attractive. Probably the most attractive male quality for a woman. If you talk dirty to a woman in bed, this is one of the most effective ways to demonstrate your gross male dominance.

Even the most conservative women I know love to talk dirty in bed; this is because women love to show up as women in public while enjoying their wild and secret sex lives. This contrast is hot for a woman.

General Rules for Dirty Talk

Whatever you say in the room stays there. While you can say dominant things in the bedroom, your wife will only allow that when understood, calling her dirty names and saying bad things is only appropriate in the bedroom context. If you treat her like a tramp outside the bedroom, your days of dirty talk are over.

Use as a spice, not as a main dish. Dirty Talks are not so much about what you say, but about who you are. It is a by-product of being an alpha male.

If you are attached to it, she will see through your cunning and have the opposite effect. Instead, be obsessed with being the MAN. Relax and let the dirty words come the way they should.

Dominant tone. Speak like a dominant caveman claiming his wife. It's one of the times in life that this is appropriate, so relax and enjoy it.

Women want to submit to a strong man, not a weak man. Your voice is the most obvious gift of how strong you are as a man. Add base to your voice and speak deliberately.

Don't forget to dominate her physically. If you bold to use dirty words, you must also have physical behavior that reflects that behavior. Don't be afraid to pull her hair out a little, spank her or throw her over your shoulder and go to the bedroom.

This warm/cold behavior strongly pushes on her emotional buttons, and the effect of the dirty talk is amplified.

Don't just say, "You're a dirty bitch, I want to damn you!" saying, "My darling, you smell so sweet" while caressing her gently ... then press her firmly against the wall and say, "I should punish you for being so hot!" The contrast shocked her into deep arousal.

Secret About Women, Sex and Dirty Talk in The Bedroom

Here's A Secret You Must Know About Women...

The truth is that when you talk dirty and do it right, you drive your wife crazy and give her the best orgasms of her life (much better than what you can do with "physical" techniques).

Dirty talk indeed improves the physical techniques you use in the bedroom.

A secret about women, sex, and dirty talk in the bedroom is revealed.

First, let's talk about the two types of women you can choose to have sex with:

Promiscuous Women

Promiscuous women sleep with many men. Many men think that these women are completely sexual. The truth is, promiscuous women rarely like sex. So why do they sleep with so many men?

The answer is that promiscuous women sleep and have a lot of sex because they want to make themselves feel better. The truth is, it never works. But that's why they do it - they're approval seekers. In other words, they are looking for validation.

High-quality women

High-quality women only sleep with the right man. They can go without sex for several months and then boom- they meet the good man where they are entirely comfortable and attracted, and they always want sex.

These women are extremely sexual and love sex, but they only want great sex.

High-quality women are generally intelligent, resourceful, creative, and adventurous.

Note that there are other types of women, but these are the two main types.

So now that you know the two main types of women, let's talk about this secret.

The secret is that if you want to have good sex and want a woman who does all the naughty things you want to do in the bedroom while responding exceptionally well to your dirty talk, you have to choose a high-quality woman.

Dirty talks are lost to promiscuous women. They don't really like sex and have "problems," they have to solve their problem before they can enjoy sex for what it is - instead of making it a validation game.

On the other hand, the more a woman has a high quality- the more she will love your dirty talk. A woman of high quality will demand dirty talk because she needs a man who can stimulate her mind rather than just her body.

The bottom line is that if you want to give a woman sexual pleasure beyond her wildest dreams and orgasms that make her scream your name, you have to choose a woman of high quality and talk dirty in the bedroom.

All real men talk dirty in the bedroom and choose their wives carefully.

Dirty Talk and What to Say

Dirty talk and what to say in dirty talk doesn't have to be rubbish talk like something you'd hear in a porn movie. If you want to talk dirty, there are tips for you. First of all, know that one of the best ways to talk dirty is to ask what you want.

Instead of just moaning and groaning in bed, tell your husband simple things like "faster," "harder," or "deeper." This allows him to vocally know what you like and how you want it without saying too much and saving you from uncomfortable moments.

Once you feel comfortable practicing the dirty talk above, you can move on to the next step to add praise somewhere along the line.

An example of this would be "Oh, yes! Right There, that is the place, do it faster" this simple phrase is naughty but not at the level you would hear in porn. If you say it in your most sensual voice, it will be very sexy, and your dirty talk will please his ears.

Try to ease into talking dirty gradually instead of jumping straight in with something shocking - it's a good idea to test the water first; otherwise, you could confuse or push your partner away.

Introducing a few 'construction' phrases is an excellent place to start and help you get into the flow of things before having sex.

Once you get started and feel like your partner responds well to what you say, you can get more adventurous and experiment with different words and phrases to see how they feel.

Let's take a look at some Dirty talk phrases you can try before and during sex with your partner:

Before Sex

• I need you now

- I am so excited to think about you

- I can't wait to feel you inside me

- I want to kiss you everywhere

- You can do whatever you want with me tonight

- I can't wait until the two of us are alone so that I get you naked

- I imagine us naked together right now

- I just had the most fantastic flashback from last night

- Do you want to have an evening early tonight?

- "I feel so weak and excited at the same time when I am in your arms."

- "I want to offer you the best oral sex you've ever had."

- "I can't wait until the two of us are alone so I can surprise you.

- "I want to tie you up later and have my way with you."

• "Feeling you above me and in control is the hottest thing ever!"

• "I thought about you last night before you fell asleep ..."

• "I love the way you look at me when we're together, it's so hot!"

During Sex

• You feel so great

• I love how thick/wet/soft you feel now

• Never stop what you are doing

• It is the best feeling ever

• You turn me on so much

• I want you to take control of me

• I want to taste you

• I want you to kiss/lick me there/ here

- "Lie down and let me take care of things."

- "I like to feel you in my hands!"

- "Continue, continue!"

- "I like the way you taste."

- "Don't stop; it's so good!"

- "You dominating me is such a turn on."

- "I want you to take control of me."

- "Stop talking, and just do me!"

- "I never want you to stop; it's such good."

- "I want you to end where you want."

If you want to deliver these lines efficiently, consider these things:

The Tone of Your Voice

Sometimes a deep, moving tone is ideal for creating and reminding you of sexual tension, while other times, a more aroused and varied tone is perfect for arousing him.

How Fast You Speak

Speaking slowly is almost always more powerful than speaking quickly when talking dirty.

Chapter 6.
Setting the Mood with Confidence

When talking erotically with your partner, there is a certain level of intimacy that must be achieved. This intimacy is very important, because otherwise, your words will fall flat and will be deemed almost ridiculous in away.

You have to set the mood and make sure that you maintain it as well. You can do this in several ways, but you cannot set the mood without first gaining confidence.

Why Is Confidence Important?

If you do not have confidence, it can bring an air of uncertainty to your bedroom endeavors. This is something that you would find yourself struggling to overcome.

First impressions are everything, and if you are not confident the first time you try to introduce erotic conversation, you could turn your partner off from it for a long time.

Confidence is the foundation for anything in life. If you want to reach any of your goals, confidence will get you farther than even knowledge, because you will not constantly second guess yourself.

Doing this can lead to many different mistakes that will cause you possibly not to achieve your goal. You must have confidence when you are trying to dirty talk. It will make your words appear to come out effortlessly and to help you encourage your partner to join in.

When you seem confident, your partner will use your confidence to help build theirs.

Confidence is sexy. It is the drive behind what gets the libido up and running. You have to be able to have confidence for dirty talk, because it is all about being sexy, and you cannot pull off sexy without confidence.

No confidence means an ineffective attempt at wooing your partner with words.

Life becomes easier to handle. The less you try to tear yourself down, the more you love yourself. This makes it easier to face every day because you are not your own worst enemy. When you genuinely believe in yourself, you can find a lot more to enjoy in life. This makes life a lot easier to look forward to.

You won't rely on outside validation. The most attractive traits in a person is their ability to be sure of themselves. These people do not need validation from others and find themselves quite appealing in their rights. They feel this way without being overly cocky, and they have a great balance of self-assurance.

You will not be afraid of the good things in life. By not being afraid of these things, you will be less likely to sabotage your attempts to find happiness, because you will know that you deserve them.

This helps in relationships because you will not try to push the other person away and will want to bring them closer. You will be confident when you find the right person and will want to show them the real you, rather than trying to get them to tell you who to be.

Why Might Confidence Be Lacking?

Some people just seem to ooze confidence in everything that they do. They feel as if they are meant to do whatever it is they set their mind to. When they go for something, it just seems to fall in their lap. You may not have this much confidence, and that is okay. The important question is why you feel that way.

Insecurities run rampant in the world. Some people are told from a young age that they are not good enough, and it is engrained in their minds. The entire world could tell them that they are good enough for some people, but it just takes one trusted person to tell them that they aren't to wreck their self-confidence. Whatever the reason, not having confidence can mean disaster for you.

Some people seem to feel like they must be perfect at everything, including looks to have confidence. This is not the truth. No one is perfect at everything, and trying to be can leave you a nervous wreck.

This is not a good way to introduce dirty talk. You must go in having the confidence to cover up any words that may not have been phrased properly. You must have confidence so that you are not dissuaded when it doesn't go perfectly, because there will be those days.

Confidence is something that not everyone has naturally, and that is okay. There is a way to build your confidence, even if you do not seem to have any. You just have to make sure that you follow through with all of these steps. When you are trying to build your confidence, it is key to remember that it does not always happen in one day, and you have to work hard at it, and on yourself as well.

You can't give up just because you do not find yourself the best in the world after trying for a day or two to build your confidence. It does not work like that, and that can cause many people to give up because they want the easy way out.

Giving up would be social torture to yourself. You have to keep working on it to make yourself a better person and a better partner. No one wants to constantly have to reassure their partner that they find them attractive and sexy. You have to be able to assure yourself because you want people to want you, not feel like they have to want you.

If you give up, you could find yourself in a bit of a tough spot and not achieve what you wanted to achieve in your goals of becoming a more open person in the bedroom. You must have confidence.

The Steps to Gaining Confidence

Confidence generally takes some work, so do not worry if you are not the most confident person in the world. You can learn how to gain confidence in yourself with these steps. These steps are designed to help even the most self-conscious gain enough confidence to be more adventurous in the bedroom.

The first step to gaining confidence is to simply fake it. That's right, pretending that you have confidence will eventually trick your brain into thinking that you are confident. This will make it simpler to build up your real confidence.

When you fake confidence, it will have other people noticing that you seem surer of yourself. This validation will show you that it works. When you look good, you feel better, and that is the mentality that is faking it uses.

It may seem silly, but "fake it till you make it" is not a saying for no reason. It applies here too. Faking it does not necessarily mean acting like the jock in a cheesy nineties movie; it simply means believing in yourself a little more, or at least acting as you do.

Setting the mood

It is important to light the mood with your partner. You have to make sure that you are making them comfortable and turning them on simultaneously. There are several things that you can do to set the mood. The first is communication.

Communication

Communication will open the door to being able to dirty talk with your partner. If you can communicate about anything with your partner, you will be able to set the mood a lot easier because you can both talk about whether it is the right time to engage in sexual conversation. If you are not able to communicate, sometimes one of you may not be in the mood, and setting the mood will be futile because it will feel forced.

It is true. Communication is the key to any relationship. Especially when it comes to something like Kamasutra, it is the duty of each partner to ensure that they satisfy their lover, but they also must let their lover know how they are feeling.

Humans are not minded readers and often do not know what you are thinking. You have to be honest with your partner and allow your partner to be open with you; otherwise, you will have some serious issues. Often, people are not open because their partners shut them down and get angry at criticism, so they feel that they are not able to be open. You have to encourage communication both in and out of the bedroom.

In the bedroom, make your partner feel comfortable with vocalization. If they are nervous, let them know that it is not silly, and you like knowing that what you are doing feels good, or if it doesn't feel good, you want to know so that you can make the proper adjustments. You should also lead by example. A lot of times, one partner is very vocal, while the other is silent, you should both be vocal. Do not be afraid of shouting or screaming in pleasure.

Also, do not be afraid to tell your partner what doesn't feel good. You can make it less harsh by asking them to change something nicely, rather than saying that hurts. This way, there is no killing of the mood.

You also need communication in your everyday life as well. When your partner upsets you, you should tell them rather than bottling it until it becomes a fight. You should also tell them if they are doing something you like. Too often in the real world, everyone talks about what they don't like, but no one talks about what they do like. Yet in the bedroom, it is the opposite. You should find a balance in both.

Communication is a necessary part of your everyday life. Even if it is just talking about your day. Many relationships fail because there is not enough communication to keep the passion alive. You want to tell your partner everything. When they ask how your day was, it is because they want to know. They do not want a one-word answer, such as "good." When they ask you, be free with the information. Tell them every little boring detail and then ask them about their day. Revel in what they are saying to you, even if the words are unimportant. Your lover will be happy knowing that you want to know about it, even if they had a really boring day. Things like that are the little things that make the world go round and truly make a relationship work. Communication is a show of love, and it will help keep your love strong. Use it to its fullest power.

Making Your Partner Comfortable

The biggest way to get your partner comfortable is communication. However, there is one other thing you can do to help get in the mood.

Make them feel good about themselves. Help boost your partner's self-confidence. This will help relax them and allow them to relax, knowing you find them as attractive as they feel they need to be to reciprocate. To do this, you simply have to compliment them.

Compliment Them

A lot of the time, being self-conscious is a big problem. People are so caught up in self-image that it is hard to be confident in your skin. A lot of that has to do with the way bodies are portrayed in the media. The world has this idea of perfection and expects everyone to reach it.

Even if your partner does not say it out loud, chances are, they have a poor self-image. Everyone struggles with some form of insecurity, and there are not enough compliments going around in the world these days.

Find five things about your partner that you like visually and five things about them that you like outside of their physical appearance. Throughout the day, compliment them on these things.

Make sure they understand that your compliments are sincere. It is best to look them in the eyes when you compliment them. Compliments will make them feel like they are on top of the world.

Do not overdo the compliments, though, because they can begin to feel insincere. Make them heartfelt and true. Do not use them just to get ready for sex. You should be complimenting your partner regularly.

Build up their self-esteem so that they feel like they are powerful.

You may be surprised at the wild side they could unleash when they feel like they are truly good for you. It is quite a sight to behold.

Chapter 7.
Dirty Talk and Fantasies

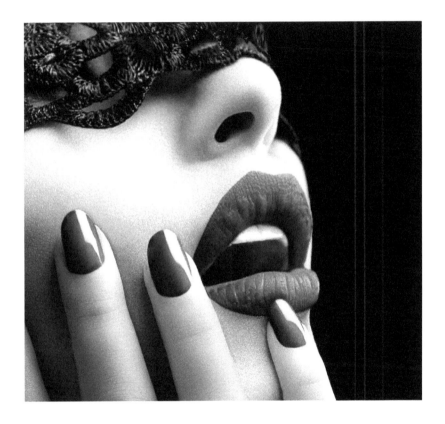

Most people have some kind of fantasy or kink, even if they've never tried it or spoken of it. We're often told our fantasies are gross or bad because of our backgrounds and other experiences, so we repress them.

However, surveys have shown that both men and women have some things they want to try, so if you're wondering about your partner, odds are they have a secret. By expressing your desires for a role-play, you are permitting them to open up, too.

How to Bring It Up

Bringing up a sexual fantasy isn't too different from bringing up dirty talk in general. Depending on the nature of the fantasy, however, you might be feeling more anxious. Maybe you anticipate your partner being very surprised by this idea and uncertain.

Conclusion this means you should only bring it up when it's just you two, in private, and feel emotionally close and safe. After sex is a very good time, because sexy stuff is already on both your minds, and it won't be as jarring for your partner.

 Another example of a good time is watching a TV show or movie and a couple onscreen role-plays. The idea is already floating in the air, so bringing it up won't seem so random or startling. Once the time is right, what do you say? Here are some ideas:

(After watching a movie/show with role-playing): Do you think that looks like it could be fun?

(After watching a movie/show with role-playing): I've always wanted to try role-playing. Is that something you would be interested in?

(After sex): Next time, there's something new I want to try, if that's okay. (Describe what you want.)

(After sex): Want to hear about my ultimate sexual fantasy?

(After sex): Can I tell you about something I've always wanted to try?

Refer to a Movie or Book

If you find it challenging to describe your fantasy in your own words, you can show your partner what you mean by using porn (if they're cool with it), reading erotic lit, or previewing a costume or toy.

Many sexual fantasies come from porn, and there's no clearer way of showing your partner what you like than by pointing them to a reenactment. If you're both comfortable with it, watching the video together can be a very intimate experience or watch it by themselves.

Maybe your fantasy originates from a book, or there's a book that simply demonstrates the fantasy really well. Read it out loud to your partner if you want, or if you feel awkward doing that, have them read it silently.

Both porn and/or erotica are great ways to clarify what exactly your fantasy is and gives your partner a good idea of the kinds of words/phrases you respond to.

Show-and-Tell Some Items Related to Your Fantasy

If you know your partner responds best to visuals, you can show off an outfit or demonstrate a toy for them. If they aren't into porn, this is an especially helpful idea because they get to see you acting out what you want.

Tell them to sit back and take it easy while you model your maid/cop/professor/astronaut/whatever costume.

Talk to them as if you were that character, so they get a clear idea of what excites you. Show them the toy and explain (sensually, of course) how to use it. If your fantasy doesn't involve a costume or accessories - maybe you want to have sex in a certain location - set the scene with your words or even take them there, pointing out where exactly you would like to get busy.

Easing into Role-Playing

Even if you feel comfortable with regular dirty talk, using it while role-playing can be tricky at first.

You're using your imagination a lot more because you aren't just describing what you're feeling in the moment; you're embodying a character or personality that might be very different from your own.

For example, being dominated is a common fantasy for women, and their partners might feel uncertain about how far they should go. Even if an extreme persona isn't part of the fantasy, there's still anxiety about convincing enough or just sounding dumb. Here are some ways to melt away anxieties and get comfortable with fantasy:

Talk it out

Before you dress up or break out the handcuffs or whatever it is you're into, it's a good idea to just sit down and talk through the fantasy, play-by-play. Often, the dirty talk is the most important part of the experience, especially if the fantasy is something the couple doesn't want to do (say, a threesome in the basement of an Italian castle); they just want to imagine it.

Get comfortable and set the scene. Say what you want to do and what you want your partner to do. Go back and forth, describing the sex.

If you describe a scenario that you plan on actually acting out at some point, be sure to only describe what you would be comfortable doing or saying. If you're narrating a more extreme scene, you would never be a part of real life, be sure your partner knows that. Ask questions to prompt your partner, like:

(Cop/criminal fantasy) "I'm holding the handcuffs and teasing you about arresting me. What do you do?"

(Dominating fantasy) "I've been a bad boy/girl. How are you going to punish me?"

(Cheating or threesome fantasy) "You see me across the room, whispering in a gorgeous woman/man's ear and playing with their hair. What do you want to do?"

(School or workplace fantasy) "You're seeing me for the first time; I'm a new student/coworker/professor/doctor/nurse/etc. What do you notice first, and what kind of dirty thoughts cross your mind?"

(Extreme environments/apocalypse fantasy) "It's so hot here in the desert, and I'm begging you for your canteen. What are you going to make me do to get it?"

(Extreme environments/snowed in fantasy) "We're all alone here in this freezing cabin, and no help can make it through the snow for hours. What should we do to keep warm?"

Keep it simple

Playing out your fantasies doesn't need to be complicated. Sometimes just an outfit or a toy is all you need to create a sexy illusion. Your dirty talk can be the same as always if that's what you want.

If you want to spice it up a bit and get more specific, try saying just one dirty thing relevant to the fantasy per sex session. As an example, let's say you're pretending you're a virgin. Slip in, "I can't believe it feels this good my first time." Maybe you're a student seducing their professor, so say something like, "I bet

I'm going to get an A on tomorrow's test." As you get more comfortable, you can start talking more.

Establish clear boundaries

If you're getting into role-playing, you should have a safe word. That isn't something limited to the pros. Since role-playing is all about pretending, this safe word will snap both of you back out of it, so you know when things are real, and you are yourselves again.

Communicate beforehand about the words/phrases you don't want at all included in your role play. Maybe you're usually more refined and want to feel dirtier during sex, so words like "slut" and "whore" are welcome during the fantasy, but you draw the line at "cunt." Maybe you are the partner being asked to call your lover a word you can't bear to slip past your lips, even when you're pretending to be someone else.

Let your partner know beforehand. Boundaries might change over time; they might not - both are perfectly fine.

Dirty Talk Ideas for Different Fantasy Scenarios

You're playing out your fantasy in a comfortable way and want to amp things up with some dirty talk. As we mentioned before, you don't have to say a lot or even say things specific to that role-play, but odds are it will help keep you at the moment and strengthen the fantasy. It would be impossible to cover every scenario, but here are some common fantasies and ideas on what to say:

Virgin + bad boy/girl

"I've been warned about guys/girls like you."

"I know I shouldn't do this, but I can't help myself."

"I'm going to make your first time unforgettable."

"Be gentle; it's my first time."

"I'm not sure how to do this. Can you show me?"

"Don't worry about anything; I'll take good care of you."

Cop + criminal

"I've been very bad, officer. What are you going to do to me?"

"I've always had a thing for men/women in uniform."

"That uniform looks tight, officer. Maybe you could loosen up a little?"

"I'm going to need to perform a strip search."

"I'm going to need to handcuff you."

"If you do something for me, I may let you go with just a warning."

Boss + employee

"Is there anything I can do to improve this performance review?"

"If you're not busy, I'd like to talk about that raise."

"I'm not so sure that skirt/blouse is appropriate for the workplace."

"I keep getting fired because I can't help sleeping with/fucking the boss."

"I hope you're not in the habit of fucking your employees, or I'm going to get jealous."

Student + teacher

"I know you're the professor, but I think there are a few things I could teach you."

"I hope you're a lot better at fucking/sucking/other sex acts than you are at math/English/science/subject of your choice."

"If I don't get an A on the next test, I think I'm going to need extra help."

"You did very poorly on that last assignment, so I think you could benefit from a little one-on-one time."

"That lecture was really interesting. Can we talk about it more alone in your office?"

"Congratulations on doing so well on that test. I have an idea about how we should celebrate."

Doctor/nurse + patient

"It's time for your physical."

"I'm going to need to take a real close look at you."

"Well, you look like you're in perfect shape. Let's make sure everything works."

"I'm having trouble with these buttons/zippers. Can you help me?"

"I've been having trouble getting hard/getting wet/getting aroused. Any ideas on how to fix that?"

"When I touch you here, do you feel any pain or something else?"

"It's time for your sponge bath. It looks like you're going to need a lot of soaping up."

Strangers/one-night stand

"You must be new in town; I would remember an ass/body/face like yours."

"I'm only in the city for tonight. What's something fun and exciting I could do to remember my visit?"

"I love that shirt/skirt/another article of clothing, but I'm curious about what's underneath."

"It's still early - want to come back to my place?"

"I never do this, but you're so sexy, I just can't help myself."

"No names, just kiss/suck/fuck me."

Royalty + servant

"I'll do whatever you wish, my queen/king."

"I'm at your command."

"I'm here to serve you."

"Your queen/king requires your services."

"Strip for your queen/king."

"Obey me."

"Worship your queen/king."

Masseuse + client

"You've got a lot of tension down here."

"I think I know just how to end this massage."

"I didn't think a woman/man this beautiful/handsome/sexy/hot would ever have their hands all over me."

"If you want an extra tip, I have an idea of how you could earn it."

"I'm going to have to ask my assistant to cancel the rest of my appointments. I think we're going to be here a while."

"I know I shouldn't say this, but I don't think I've ever felt a body this hard/muscled/sleek/smooth/perfect before."

Escort + client

"Can you go over what services you're offering tonight?"

"Kiss me as you mean, I want to feel like I'm getting my money's worth."

"It's been a long time since someone worked my body like that."

"I have a feeling you're going to like what I'm offering."

"You're so hot; you're making my job easy."

"You're going to get your money's worth tonight."

Dominatrix + client

"I've been naughty, and I need my master/mistress to punish me."

"I'll do anything you want."

"Don't talk unless I say you can talk."

"Get on your knees."

"I'm in charge now, so you better pay attention."

"You can't cum until I give you permission."

Celebrity + roadie/groupie

"I brought the stuff you wanted from the van. Is there anything else I can do for you?"

"I can't believe I'm actually meeting you. There's this one thing I always promised myself I would do."

"You must be so lonely always on tour, but you don't have to be alone tonight."

"You've been so helpful on the road, and I know just how to thank you."

"I saw you in the front row and knew right away that I had to have you."

"This was my last show on this tour. Any ideas on how to make it the most memorable one ever?"

Chapter 8.
Dirty Talk During the Deed

Desiring dirty talk during sex is very common for both men and women, but how do you do it? Maybe you've gotten good at sexting and building anticipation, but the thought of translating that into spoken words is intimidating. You have to think about your tone of voice, nicknames and phrases to use, and more. This chapter explores the different types of during-sex dirty talk, ideas for what to say, and how to continue dirty talk through the post-coital glow.

The Three Most Arousing Dirty-Talk Techniques

As we've said before, and talk about the sex as you have it is dirty talk, but there are three specific techniques you can use to fan the flames: describing what you're feeling, taking charge, and redirecting to sexy stuff you like:

Describing what you feel

One of the easiest ways to dirty talk is to just narrate what you're feeling in the moment. Feeling a cool tingle or throb? Tell your partner. It heightens the experience for both you and your partner when you share what's going on, and it lets them know things are going well.

When you start getting close to orgasm, keep the talk going all the way through, if you can. It turns up the heat and gets your partner excited. Depending on where you are in your dirty talk journey, you can be as general or specific as you want:

"I don't want to stop kissing you."

"My legs feel like jelly right now."

"I can't get enough of you."

"I feel so close to you."

"That thing you're doing with your tongue is driving me crazy."

"You're so good with your hands."

"You feel so big inside me."

"I love being so deep inside you."

"I'm so close. I can't stand it."

"I'm about to cum."

Taking charge

Being bossy is both sexy and gets you what you want. Both men and women often like to be dominated and told what to do, so this is the perfect dirty talk style. Be direct with your words. If your partner wants you to be more aggressive physically, as well, go for it, but unless that's an explicit desire that you're sure about, just be bossy with your voice. Here are some ideas:

"I want you right now."

"Kiss me as you mean it."

"I want your mouth on me."

"I want your tongue in me."

"Pull my hair."

"Flip me over and do me from behind."

"Pin my arms over my head."

"I want to get on top."

"Spank me."

"Ride me fast and slow/hard and easy."

"Look at me/don't look at me."

"Say my name."

"Cum for me."

Redirecting

Using dirty talk to redirect your partner is similar to taking charge. Still, it's specifically for when they're doing something you aren't really feeling or they're not quite nailing a certain technique. This is common during oral sex, which can be tricky for many people, especially if they're new to giving it. Instead of just saying, "Don't do that," which isn't very encouraging, you're giving them something else to do that you do like, using your sexy voice. When they're doing something oh-so-right, don't forget to affirm that, too.

"Slower."

"Harder."

"Faster."

"Gently."

"Deeper."

"Hold me tighter."

"Can you use your tongue?"

"Higher."

"Lower."

"I'm ready for you."

"Just like that."

"More."

"Don't stop."

What if the Dirty Talk Isn't Going Well?

Dirty talk can be awkward, especially when you're just starting. What if you're having sex and trying out some new words and phrases, and they just aren't landing? Maybe your partner isn't responding, or you just feel uncomfortable. Don't worry!

You can make things much easier by remembering you don't need a huge dictionary of dirty things to say, and you don't have to be constantly talking. This is an example of quality over quantity. Only saying a few dirty phrases per sexy time isn't a failure if that's where your comfort level is. Forcing more will be awkward and not fun.

Are you worried that you always say the same things? Your partner isn't going to care if you fall back on classics like, "This is amazing," "I love feeling you inside me/being inside you," or "I can't get enough of you right now." If those are the genuine things you feel most comfortable saying, your partner will hear the passion and earnestness in your voice.

Also, as a note, if your partner isn't responding the way you expected, it doesn't mean they aren't enjoying the dirty talk.

Maybe they are feeling self-conscious and don't know what to say back to you. After sex, ask them what they were feeling and if having them respond verbally is important, let them know.

If you are the partner who isn't talking much, but want to let your partner know how much you're enjoying the moment, focus on sounds instead.

Moaning is always welcome, though if you know your partner wants dirty talk, consider dropping in a few swear words. These are powerful, short, and simple declarations, like "Oh, fuck," "Fuck, yeah," and so on. Phrases like, "Oh, God" will also most likely be met with enthusiasm.

Dirty Talk Over Skype

Thanks to the power of technology, you can enjoy romantic encounters over video chat services like Skype! This type of sex is especially valuable for long-distance couples or for couples where one partner travels frequently. It keeps them on the same page, sexually and emotionally. Working through the initial awkwardness and vulnerability also strengthens a couple's trust in one another. Here's how to employ dirty talk over Skype:

Prep

It's safe to say that most Skype sex isn't spontaneous. That gives you some time to prepare what the session will look like and get ready. Maybe that means picking out your favorite sexy clothing, selecting a toy and/or lube (if you're planning on pleasuring yourself), choosing a playlist, or lighting a candle.

It's also the time to think about what you're going to say. Are you going to focus on describing what you're doing to yourself or narrate what you would do to your partner if you were together? Is there a particular pet name your partner likes? A phrase? Putting in the effort will make the Skype sex way hotter and more fun.

Treat it Like a Real Date

Making sure you won't be interrupted, especially crucial if you have kids or roommates. Can you even imagine how awkward it would be for everyone? Ideally, you are alone in the house with a few hours to spare. The door and windows are closed, and you're feeling comfortable.

Now, treat the Skype date like a real date. Wear what you would wear when you're ready for a sexy evening in person.

Focus all your attention on your partner, so put away the phone, turn off the TV, and close any other browser tabs. Imagine your partner is the only other person in the world right now.

Describe what you're doing (and what you wish you were doing)

Your voice is very important. Since your partner can't touch you, it's the most intimate connection. They can also see you, which helps, but there's something about a sensual tone that gets the blood pumping. What are some specific things you could say?

"You look so hot right now; there are so many things I want to do to you."

"Are you ready for me to take off my clothes?"

"I'm so wet right now."

"I'm so hard right now."

"I'm kissing your neck, behind your ear, and gripping your hair hard."

"I can feel you stroking me up and down."

"I'm imagining that you're licking me right now."

"I wish I could feel you inside me/I wish I was inside you."

"I'm thinking about you plowing/doing/fucking me so hard right now."

Lots of sounds like moans and heavy breathing are great accompaniments to dirty talk over Skype. They will instantly snap you into a sexy mindset.

If you aren't sure what to say, you can always read some erotica out loud. If you like to write, you can even write your dirty talk beforehand and read it, so it's original, and your partner knows it came from your mind.

Dirty Talk After Sex

Dirty talk doesn't have to stop once the sex is over. It's a great way to keep intimacy and communication going and provide feedback on what you liked. It's also a good time to bring up things you would like to try the next time things get hot and heavy. Here are some examples:

"I'm still weak in the knees."

"My head is still spinning."

"I'm not sure I can stand for a while."

"I loved those sounds you were making."

"It was so sexy when you... (said/did this particular thing.)"

"Mmm, I love that I can still taste you."

"We have to do that (the thing you liked) next time."

"I'm going to be thinking about that all day tomorrow."

"I wish we could just stay here like this forever."

What Not to Do

We've talked about dirty talk techniques and given you some examples, but is there anything you should not do when trying it out with your partner? There are three main rules to follow:

Don't Laugh at Your Partner

Dirty talk can be awkward, especially when it's brand-new. You may feel relatively comfortable with your tone and words, but your partner may still be getting used to it. They may come up with something cheesy or funny, and you're tempted to chuckle. Resist.

Laughing will make your partner feel dumb, and they'll clam up. They might not want to try dirty talk ever again. Instead of laughing, suggest other things they could say or a name you like, so they can try something else.

Don't Say Things You're Not Comfortable With

As you read about dirty talk and start experimenting, you might bump up against words or phrases you don't like. However, your partner might respond to them in a positive way.

Maybe you hate calling your partner a "bitch," but they like it, and they want you to get even more aggressive. It can be tempting to not talk about how uncomfortable you are because your partner is happy. This can be very harmful to your relationship. You'll feel false or worse. Because you're so uncomfortable, you won't be able to fully enjoy the sex and your partner, and that's bad for both of you. Talk to them. You can find a compromise.

Don't Rush in

Dirty talk has many layers and tones. Most people like to ease into it, even if they know how extreme they would like to go. This is a good idea because it lets both you and your partner discover your limits and what you like.

Rushing in can be overwhelming and create uncomfortable or even disturbing situations that paint dirty talk in a bad light. Being a bit cautious and careful is especially important if you and your partner have not been together very long.

You're still establishing trust. Just take things slow. It's about the fun and excitement of going on the journey and not reaching a set destination.

What About Dirty Talk and Role-Playing?

As you were reading this chapter, you might have wondered why we weren't bringing up role-playing. Dirty talk is an essential part of fantasy and role-play, though it can take a while to get comfortable if it's unfamiliar to you.

Main Takeaways

There are three very arousing types of dirty talk during sex: describing what you're feeling, telling your partner exactly what you want, and redirecting your partner to try something else.

If you feel awkward trying dirty talk and it doesn't seem to be going well, you can fall back on words or phrases you are comfortable with or focus on making sounds instead. You don't need to break out something fresh every time.

To have good Skype sex, have an idea about what you're going to say and do, and treat the event like a real date. If you're pleasuring yourself, be sure to describe what you're doing for your partner and detail what you wish you could do to them.

Dirty talk can also be a part of your after-sex experience. Talk about what you liked, what you want to try next time, and just enjoy each other.

The only things you should not do when dirty talking are laughing at what your partner says, saying things you aren't comfortable with, and rushing the process. These three no-no's paint dirty talk in a negative light.

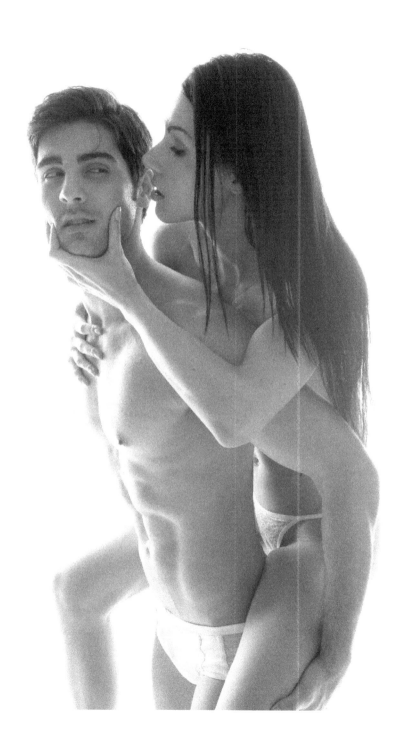

Conclusion

It may start slow and bumpy in the beginning, but keep practicing until you get there.

Getting over the shyness in the initial stage is probably the hardest bit.

Once you've over that hump, though, verbalizing your raw passion and desire for your lover is going to roll smoothly off the tongue.

Don't forget to keep expanding your erotic vocabulary, either.

Incorporate as many sexy, seductive phrases into your routine, and you'll become a pro at this in no time.

That being said, try to avoid the mistake of memorizing all the phrases you have learned in this book.

These are meant to serve as a point of reference, and that's it.

CPSIA information can be obtained
at www.ICGtesting.com
Printed in the USA
BVHW040256200122
626621BV00014B/1349